Table of Contents

1. Understanding Low t Is It Really?
2. Recognizing the Signs – Symptoms and Diagnosis
3. Why Testosterone Levels Decline – Causes and Risk Factors
4. Natural Ways to Boost Testosterone – Lifestyle, Diet, and Self-Care
5. Medical Treatments for Low Testosterone – What Works and What to Avoid
6. Regaining Vitality – A Long-Term Plan for Optimal Testosterone

Chapter 1: Understanding Low Testosterone – What Is It Really?

Testosterone's Role in Men's Health

Testosterone is often thought of as the defining male hormone, but its influence extends far beyond muscle growth and libido. It is the driving force behind **energy levels, mood stability, fat metabolism, cognitive sharpness, and overall physical strength**. Produced primarily in the testes, with a small amount from the adrenal glands, testosterone plays a key role in **maintaining muscle mass, bone density, red blood cell production, and reproductive health**. When levels are balanced, men experience **strong motivation, steady energy, and a robust sense of well-being**. When levels drop, everything changes.

Despite its importance, testosterone is often overlooked until symptoms of deficiency begin to appear. Men who experience chronic fatigue, loss of strength, mental fog, or diminishing confidence may not immediately connect these changes to hormones. Yet, testosterone impacts nearly every system in the body, from the brain to the cardiovascular system. Without adequate levels, **both physical and mental performance suffer**, often leading to frustration and confusion.

Why Testosterone is Called the "Male Vitality Hormone"

Testosterone is not just about masculinity—it is about **vitality, drive, and resilience**. It influences **metabolism, muscle preservation, and even how men respond to challenges**. Healthy levels contribute to:

Steady motivation and mental clarity.
A leaner body composition with easier muscle maintenance.
A stronger heart and more efficient oxygen transport.
Healthy sleep cycles that support recovery and immune function.
A positive mood and greater resistance to stress.
Many men assume that feeling sluggish, gaining weight, or losing interest in activities is a natural part of aging. While some decline

in testosterone is expected over time, **a significant drop can lead to noticeable and unnecessary struggles**. Understanding what testosterone does—and how to maintain optimal levels—can help prevent these changes from taking control.

What Happens When Testosterone Levels Drop?

A decline in testosterone doesn't happen overnight. It is often **gradual and easy to dismiss at first**, making it one of the most overlooked causes of physical and mental changes in men. Many assume that feeling constantly tired, unmotivated, or struggling with weight gain is just part of getting older. But when testosterone drops **below optimal levels**, the effects can reach every part of life—**energy, strength, mental clarity, and even emotional resilience**.

One of the first signs of Low-T is **fatigue that doesn't go away with rest**. Unlike normal tiredness from a long day, testosterone-related fatigue feels **unrelenting, draining, and hard to shake**. Even after a full night's sleep, men with low testosterone often wake up feeling **just as exhausted as they did the night before**. This lack of energy is accompanied by a **loss of motivation**, making even simple tasks feel overwhelming.

Another common sign is **a noticeable drop in muscle mass and an increase in body fat**, especially around the abdomen. Since testosterone is responsible for **muscle maintenance and fat metabolism**, low levels make it harder to build strength and easier to gain weight. Even men who continue working out may find that **their body is not responding the way it used to**.

The Mental and Emotional Toll of Low Testosterone

While most people associate testosterone with **physical strength**, its impact on mental health is just as significant. Low-T often leads to **brain fog, difficulty concentrating, and forgetfulness**, making it harder to stay sharp and focused. Many men report feeling like **they're losing their edge**—struggling to stay productive at work, forgetting details more often, or feeling mentally sluggish in conversations.

The emotional effects can be just as frustrating. **Mood swings, irritability, and even depression** are common with Low-T, yet many men don't realize their hormones are to blame. **Testosterone helps regulate dopamine and serotonin**, the brain's "feel-good" chemicals. When levels drop, motivation, confidence, and emotional resilience suffer. Small setbacks start to feel overwhelming, and once-enjoyable activities lose their appeal.

Low testosterone also affects **stress response**. Men with healthy testosterone levels **recover from challenges more easily**—whether that's pushing through a tough workout, handling a demanding work project, or managing emotional stress. When testosterone is low, **stress feels heavier, anxiety becomes more frequent, and the ability to bounce back is weaker**.

The Warning Signs Many Men Overlook

Because Low-T symptoms develop gradually, many men adapt to the changes without realizing their health is declining. The most commonly ignored signs include:

- Constant fatigue, even after a full night's sleep.
- Increased belly fat and difficulty maintaining muscle.
- Brain fog, forgetfulness, and lack of focus.
- Loss of motivation and interest in things that used to bring excitement.
- Feeling emotionally drained or less confident in decision-making.
- Irritability, mood swings, or frequent frustration over small things.
- Reduced recovery after workouts or feeling weaker than before.

These symptoms are often dismissed as **aging, stress, or lack of discipline**, but the real cause is often hormonal imbalance. Understanding these warning signs is the first step toward **taking back control of energy, strength, and mental sharpness**.

The Growing Problem of Low Testosterone in Modern Men

Testosterone levels are declining across generations, and it's not just because men are getting older. Studies have shown that **average testosterone levels in men today are significantly lower than they were decades ago.** This means that many men in their 30s and 40s are experiencing symptoms of Low-T **earlier than expected**, and even younger men are being diagnosed with hormonal imbalances that used to be rare.

There are several factors contributing to this widespread decline. **Modern lifestyles, environmental toxins, and chronic stress** are all playing a role in disrupting hormone production. Unlike previous generations, men today are exposed to **endocrine-disrupting chemicals found in plastics, processed foods, and everyday household products**. These chemicals interfere with the body's ability to produce and regulate testosterone, leading to **lower levels at younger ages**.

At the same time, **sedentary lifestyles, poor sleep habits, and rising obesity rates** are making the problem worse. Testosterone thrives when the body is active, well-nourished, and properly rested. Yet, modern routines often involve **long hours sitting at desks, high stress, poor diets, and inadequate recovery**, all of which contribute to declining hormone levels.

Is Low Testosterone Just a Part of Aging?

One of the biggest misconceptions about testosterone is that its decline is **inevitable and untreatable**. While testosterone does naturally decrease with age, the rate at which it drops—and whether it leads to symptoms—varies widely. Some men maintain **healthy testosterone levels well into their 60s and 70s**, while others experience sharp declines in their 30s. The difference often comes down to **lifestyle choices, genetics, and underlying health conditions**.

Aging alone is not the reason testosterone levels are plummeting in younger men today. The real issue is that **modern habits are**

accelerating hormonal decline, making men feel older than they actually are. Symptoms of Low-T—such as chronic fatigue, stubborn weight gain, and reduced motivation—are often blamed on "just getting older," but in many cases, **they can be improved or reversed** with the right approach.

How "Normal" Is Normal? The Debate Over Testosterone Levels

Many men experiencing symptoms of Low-T get tested, only to be told their results are **within the normal range**. This can be confusing, especially when energy is low, muscle mass is decreasing, and mental sharpness is fading. The problem is that **"normal" testosterone levels vary widely**, and what is considered "normal" in a lab report is not always **optimal** for an individual's health and performance.

Doctors typically measure **total testosterone**, but this number alone does not always tell the full story. **Free testosterone—the portion of testosterone available for use in the body—is often a more accurate marker of how**

well the hormone is functioning. Some men with "normal" total testosterone still experience symptoms because their free testosterone is low due to high levels of **sex hormone-binding globulin (SHBG)**, which limits testosterone's availability.

The key takeaway is that **testosterone levels should not be assessed based on lab numbers alone**. Symptoms, lifestyle, and overall well-being **matter just as much—if not more—than what a test result says**. Many men are struggling unnecessarily simply because they have been told their levels are "fine" when, in reality, they could benefit from treatment or lifestyle changes.

Recognizing that **Low-T is not just a normal part of aging but a fixable problem** is the first step toward regaining control. With the right approach, testosterone levels can often be **optimized, leading to renewed energy, better health, and a stronger sense of well-being**.

How Low is "Low"? Understanding Testosterone Ranges

One of the most frustrating parts of dealing with low testosterone is the **confusion surrounding what's considered "normal."** Many men go to the doctor with clear symptoms of Low-T, only to be told their testosterone levels fall within the "acceptable range." But what does that actually mean?

Testosterone levels are typically measured in **nanograms per deciliter (ng/dL)** of blood. The so-called "normal" range can vary by lab, but it generally falls between **250 and 1,000 ng/dL**. That's an incredibly wide range, and what's normal for one man might be completely inadequate for another.

A young, healthy man will typically have **total testosterone levels between 600 and 1,000 ng/dL**, while anything under 300 ng/dL is often classified as Low-T. But here's where things get tricky: some men can feel fantastic at 400 ng/dL, while others experience severe fatigue and loss of motivation at the same level. That's because **total testosterone doesn't tell the whole story**.

The Difference Between Total, Free, and Bioavailable Testosterone

Total testosterone is just one measurement. More important for how a man actually feels is **free testosterone**, which represents the small portion of testosterone that is active and available for the body to use.

Much of the testosterone circulating in the blood is **bound to proteins like sex hormone-binding globulin (SHBG) and albumin**. When testosterone binds to SHBG, it becomes inactive and unavailable to cells. This means a man could have **total testosterone within the normal range but still experience Low-T symptoms if too much of it is bound to SHBG**.

That's why **free testosterone** and **bioavailable testosterone** are crucial measurements. Free testosterone makes up only about **2–3% of total testosterone**, but this is the portion that directly influences

energy, mood, libido, and muscle maintenance. Bioavailable testosterone includes free testosterone plus the fraction loosely bound to albumin, which can still be used by the body.

Some men have total testosterone levels around **500 ng/dL but feel awful because their free testosterone is too low**. Others may have a total level of **350 ng/dL but feel fine because their free testosterone is in an optimal range**. This variation is why testing **free and bioavailable testosterone, along with SHBG levels, provides a more accurate picture of hormonal health**.

Symptoms Matter More Than Lab Numbers

A man's **individual experience is more important than his lab results**. Some doctors will dismiss symptoms if a man's total testosterone is above 300 ng/dL, even though that number is on the low end of the spectrum. But a man with **chronic fatigue, brain fog, weight gain, and loss of motivation** should not be ignored just because his blood test falls within a wide reference range.

The best way to determine if Low-T is a problem is by looking at **both lab work and symptoms** together. If a man is experiencing classic signs of testosterone deficiency—**low energy, mood instability, muscle loss, and poor sleep**—then it's worth taking a deeper look at his hormone levels.

Understanding that **"low" is not just a number but a combination of lab results and how a man feels** is key. Many men go years without proper treatment simply because they were told their levels were "fine." But testosterone optimization is not about being barely within range—it's about finding the levels that allow a man to **feel his best, function optimally, and maintain long-term health**.

The Long-Term Effects of Untreated Low-T

Many men brush off symptoms of low testosterone as temporary issues—something they can push through or ignore. But untreated Low-T is more than just an inconvenience. Over time, it can lead to **serious long-term health consequences** that go far beyond energy and libido. The body relies on testosterone for a wide range of essential functions, and when levels remain low for extended periods, the risks become more severe.

One of the biggest dangers of Low-T is **accelerated muscle loss and increased fat gain**. Testosterone plays a direct role in maintaining **muscle mass, metabolism, and insulin sensitivity**. When levels drop, the body shifts toward fat storage, particularly around the **abdomen and chest**, which increases the risk of **metabolic syndrome, insulin resistance, and type 2 diabetes**. This makes weight management significantly harder, even for men who exercise regularly.

Beyond metabolism, **bone health is also affected**. Testosterone helps maintain **bone**

density and strength, and men with Low-T are at a higher risk of **osteopenia and osteoporosis**, conditions typically associated with aging women. This makes fractures and injuries more likely, particularly in later years.

Low Testosterone and Heart Health

Another major concern is the connection between **Low-T and cardiovascular disease**. While testosterone was once thought to increase heart disease risk, newer research suggests that **low levels may be the real threat**. Men with Low-T are more likely to develop **high blood pressure, elevated cholesterol, and arterial plaque buildup**, all of which contribute to heart disease.

Testosterone plays a role in **red blood cell production and circulation**, meaning that inadequate levels can result in **poor oxygen delivery to muscles and organs**, leading to chronic fatigue and decreased endurance. Some studies suggest that **men with untreated Low-T have a higher risk of heart attacks and strokes**, making hormone balance essential for long-term cardiovascular health.

The Impact on Mental and Emotional Health

Beyond the physical effects, **low testosterone significantly impacts mood, motivation, and cognitive function**. Many men with Low-T experience:

- **Depression and mood swings** that feel unexplainable.
- **Loss of drive and ambition**, making even small tasks feel overwhelming.
- **Brain fog, difficulty concentrating, and short-term memory issues**.

These mental effects are often misdiagnosed as **stress, burnout, or even clinical depression**, leading some men to be prescribed antidepressants without addressing the underlying hormonal imbalance. While mental health issues can have multiple causes, **testosterone plays a direct role in regulating dopamine and serotonin**, the brain's key mood-stabilizing chemicals.

Why Ignoring Low-T Can Lead to Bigger Problems

Because Low-T develops gradually, many men don't realize how much it's affecting them until **the symptoms become impossible to ignore**. The longer it goes untreated, the more likely it is to contribute to **chronic disease, accelerated aging, and reduced quality of life**.

Ignoring testosterone decline isn't just about accepting lower energy levels—it's about **preventing the long-term damage that can make aging harder than it needs to be**. Addressing Low-T early can **preserve muscle mass, protect heart health, stabilize mood, and improve overall longevity**.

The good news? **Low testosterone is not a life sentence.** With the right approach, it can often be **improved, managed, and even reversed**, allowing men to regain their strength, vitality, and sense of control.

Can Low Testosterone Be Reversed?

One of the biggest concerns for men facing Low-T is whether they are stuck with it forever. The good news is that **low testosterone is not always permanent**, and in many cases, it can be **improved, stabilized, or even fully reversed**. The key is identifying **what's causing the decline** and taking the right steps to restore balance.

Some cases of Low-T are temporary, triggered by **lifestyle factors, stress, poor diet, or lack of sleep**. When these issues are addressed, testosterone levels often **rebound naturally**, leading to significant improvements in energy, mood, and strength. Other cases may be linked to **underlying medical conditions or genetic factors**, requiring a combination of **natural strategies and medical intervention** for optimal results.

Understanding the **difference between temporary and permanent Low-T** is essential. Men who experience a sudden drop in testosterone due to **stress, weight gain, or medication side effects** often see improvement when these triggers are removed. However, men with **chronic conditions, pituitary dysfunction, or long-term hormonal imbalances** may require more advanced treatment options, including **testosterone replacement therapy (TRT)**.

The Natural Approach vs. Medical Intervention

For many men, improving testosterone starts with **lifestyle adjustments. Optimizing diet, increasing strength training, reducing stress, and improving sleep** can all have a powerful impact on hormone levels. Supplements such as **zinc, magnesium, vitamin D, and omega-3 fatty acids** can also support natural testosterone production.

However, some men may need **medical intervention** if natural methods don't produce results. Testosterone replacement therapy (TRT) can be a life-changing solution for men with **clinically low levels** that do not respond to lifestyle changes. Other medical options, such as **Clomid or hCG therapy**, can help boost testosterone without shutting down natural production, making them a better choice for men who still want to maintain fertility.

The most important thing is that **every man's situation is different**. What works for one person may not work for another, and the best approach is one that is **personalized, monitored, and sustainable** for long-term health.

What This Book Will Cover

This book is designed to provide a **clear, practical roadmap** for identifying and addressing Low-T. Whether testosterone decline is due to **age, lifestyle, or underlying medical conditions**, the goal is to provide **science-backed solutions that can restore energy, strength, and confidence**.

- How to **recognize the early signs of Low-T** before they get worse.
- The best ways to **naturally boost testosterone** through diet, exercise, and sleep.

- When to consider **medical treatments** and what options are available.
- How to avoid common mistakes that **sabotage hormone health**.
- Strategies for maintaining **high testosterone levels for life**.

Low testosterone does not have to define a man's future. With the right approach, it is possible to **regain strength, vitality, and mental sharpness**, allowing men to feel their best at any age.

Chapter 2: Recognizing the Signs – Symptoms and Diagnosis

The Most Common Symptoms of Low-T

Low testosterone doesn't always announce itself with dramatic changes. For many men, the symptoms develop **gradually**, making them easy to **dismiss as stress, aging, or just a rough patch in life**. However, when testosterone drops below optimal levels, certain telltale signs begin to emerge—affecting **energy, mood, body composition, and overall well-being**.

One of the first and most noticeable signs is **persistent fatigue**. This isn't the kind of tiredness that goes away after a good night's sleep. Instead, it's a **deep, lingering exhaustion that makes even simple tasks feel like a struggle**. Many men describe it as feeling "drained" all the time, no matter how much they rest.

Another common issue is **low libido and sexual dysfunction**. Testosterone plays a major role in **sexual desire, performance,** and function, so when levels dip, **interest in intimacy fades**. Some men experience **erectile difficulties**, while others simply notice **a lack of drive or enthusiasm for sex**.

At the same time, **body composition begins to shift**. Testosterone helps **maintain lean muscle mass and regulate fat distribution**, so when levels drop, many men experience **muscle loss, increased belly fat, and a softer overall appearance**. Even men who continue working out often find that **gaining muscle becomes harder and recovery takes longer**.

The Subtle But Powerful Effects on the Mind

Low testosterone doesn't just affect the body—it also has a **strong impact on mental and emotional health**. Many men with Low-T struggle with **brain fog**, making it harder to focus, recall information, or think quickly. Tasks that once felt effortless **start to feel mentally draining**, leading to frustration and self-doubt.

Mood swings and **unexplained irritability** are also common. Men with Low-T often report feeling **more easily frustrated, impatient, or emotionally flat**. Things that wouldn't have bothered them before suddenly seem overwhelming, and their ability to **handle stress diminishes**.

Perhaps most concerning is the **loss of motivation and drive**. Testosterone is closely linked to **ambition, confidence, and competitiveness**, which is why men with Low-T often feel like they've "lost their edge." The fire that once fueled their careers, hobbies, and personal goals **dims**, making it harder to stay focused and engaged.

Why Many Men Overlook These Symptoms

Because testosterone decline happens gradually, many men **don't realize how much has changed until they look back and recognize what they've lost**. They may brush off their fatigue, mood shifts, or weight gain as normal aging, failing to see that these symptoms are actually **warning signs of an underlying hormone imbalance**.

Understanding these changes is the first step toward **taking action and restoring health**. The key is **not waiting until symptoms become severe** but recognizing them early and **exploring options to bring testosterone back to optimal levels**.

The Mental and Emotional Effects of Low Testosterone

Low testosterone doesn't just affect the body—it **reshapes the mind**, often in ways that men don't immediately recognize. While physical symptoms like fatigue and muscle loss are more obvious, the **psychological effects of Low-T** can be just as disruptive, if not more so.

One of the most common yet overlooked effects is **brain fog**. Many men with Low-T describe feeling like their **mental sharpness has dulled**, making it harder to focus, recall information, and think quickly. Conversations that once felt effortless now require more effort, and staying productive at work **becomes a daily struggle**.

Alongside cognitive changes, **Low-T significantly impacts mood stability**. Testosterone helps regulate dopamine and serotonin—**the brain's key neurotransmitters for motivation, confidence, and happiness**. When testosterone levels drop, these neurotransmitters become **imbalanced**, leading to:

- **Increased irritability and frustration, even over small things**.
- **Apathy and loss of enthusiasm for once-enjoyable activities**.
- **More frequent episodes of anxiety and mood swings**.

Some men find themselves **more withdrawn and emotionally flat**, feeling disconnected from their goals, relationships, and ambitions. Others experience **a decline in self-confidence**, leading to second-guessing decisions and avoiding challenges they once tackled with ease.

How Low Testosterone Contributes to Depression and Anxiety

It's no coincidence that many men struggling with **Low-T are misdiagnosed with depression or anxiety disorders**. While mental health conditions can have multiple causes, testosterone plays a direct role in **regulating stress response and emotional resilience**.

When testosterone levels drop, stress hormones like **cortisol become more dominant**, making men feel **on edge, overwhelmed, and emotionally drained**. Even minor setbacks seem harder to deal with, and feelings of frustration or sadness become more difficult to shake.

Men with Low-T may also experience:

- **Lack of motivation and drive**, making even small tasks feel like a chore.

- **Low self-esteem and feelings of inadequacy**, leading to avoidance of challenges.
- **Disturbed sleep patterns**, worsening overall mental health.

Unfortunately, many men don't connect these symptoms to Low-T, and instead, they are often prescribed **antidepressants or anti-anxiety medications that only treat the symptoms, not the root cause**. While mental health treatment is important, addressing **hormonal balance can make a dramatic difference** in overall mood and emotional stability.

Reclaiming Mental Clarity and Emotional Strength

The good news is that these mental and emotional symptoms **are not permanent**. When testosterone is restored to optimal levels—whether naturally or through medical treatment—**mental sharpness, motivation, and confidence often return**. Many men report feeling like **a fog has lifted**, regaining their ability to think clearly, stay focused, and approach life with more resilience.

Recognizing that **Low-T is not just a physical condition but one that affects every aspect of mental and emotional well-being** is critical. Understanding these effects is the first step toward taking back control and making the changes needed to feel **strong, sharp, and driven once again**.

Physical Signs That Your Testosterone Is Too Low

While many of the early symptoms of Low-T affect energy and mood, the **physical changes** that come with declining testosterone levels can be even more noticeable. Since testosterone plays a key role in **muscle growth, fat metabolism, and overall body composition**, its decline leads to **visible shifts in strength, endurance, and appearance**.

One of the most common physical signs of Low-T is **muscle loss and increased body**

fat, particularly around the abdomen and chest. Even men who continue to exercise often notice that their **muscles feel softer, recovery takes longer, and strength gains become harder to maintain**. The reason is simple: **testosterone is essential for protein synthesis**, the process by which the body builds and repairs muscle. When levels drop, so does the body's ability to maintain lean muscle mass.

At the same time, Low-T makes it easier to **gain fat, especially in the midsection**. Testosterone naturally **keeps body fat in check by regulating insulin sensitivity and metabolism**, but when levels decline, the body becomes **less efficient at burning fat and more prone to storing it**. This can lead to the frustrating cycle of **losing muscle while gaining fat, even with a good diet and workout routine**.

The Link Between Low Testosterone and Sexual Health

One of the most well-known effects of Low-T is its **impact on sexual function**, but the way it presents can vary. While some men experience **a complete loss of interest in sex**, others still have the desire but **struggle with arousal and performance**. Testosterone is directly linked to **blood flow, sensitivity, and overall sexual function**, meaning that low levels can contribute to:

- **Erectile difficulties, even when desire is present**.
- **Reduced pleasure and sensation, making intimacy less fulfilling**.
- **Longer recovery times between sexual activity**.

Many men assume that testosterone decline is a normal part of aging, but **these symptoms don't have to be accepted as an inevitable reality**. In many cases, restoring testosterone levels—whether naturally or through medical treatment—leads to **a dramatic improvement in confidence, performance, and satisfaction**.

Other Physical Symptoms of Low-T

Beyond body composition and sexual health, **Low-T can also affect hair growth, skin health, and circulation. Some men notice **thinning body or facial hair**, while others experience **drier, less elastic skin** due to reduced collagen production. Low testosterone is also linked to **poor circulation**, which can cause **cold hands and feet, slower wound healing, and overall reduced stamina**.

These physical symptoms are important warning signs that **testosterone levels may be lower than they should be**. Because the body relies on testosterone for so many functions, ignoring these changes can lead to **more severe health issues over time**. Recognizing these signals early can be the key to **taking action before symptoms become more difficult to reverse**.

How to Get Tested for Low-T

Recognizing the symptoms of Low-T is the first step, but **getting properly tested is essential for confirming the diagnosis and determining the best course of action**. Many men go years without knowing their testosterone levels simply because they **haven't had the right blood work done**. Unfortunately, some doctors rely on outdated testing methods or dismiss concerns if total testosterone falls within a broad "normal" range. That's why knowing **which tests to ask for and how to interpret the results** is key.

The most important test for diagnosing Low-T is a **total testosterone blood test**, but this alone doesn't provide the full picture. Testosterone in the body exists in two main forms—**bound and free**. Most testosterone is bound to proteins like **sex hormone-binding globulin (SHBG) and albumin**, making it unavailable for immediate use. The **free testosterone test** measures the small percentage of testosterone that is active in the body and responsible for **muscle growth, mental clarity, libido, and energy levels**.

Key Blood Tests for Evaluating Testosterone Levels

When getting tested for Low-T, it's important to request a **comprehensive hormone panel**, which includes:

- **Total testosterone** – Measures the overall amount of testosterone in the bloodstream.
- **Free testosterone** – Indicates how much testosterone is available for immediate use.
- **SHBG (Sex Hormone-Binding Globulin)** – High SHBG levels can bind too much testosterone, making less available for the body to use.
- **Estradiol (E2)** – Testosterone naturally converts to estrogen, and excess conversion can cause hormonal imbalances.
- **LH (Luteinizing Hormone)** – Helps determine if Low-T is caused by the brain not signaling the testes to produce enough testosterone.
- **FSH (Follicle-Stimulating Hormone)** – Important for assessing sperm production and fertility concerns.

- **DHEA and DHT** – Precursors and metabolites of testosterone that help in diagnosing overall hormone function.

By evaluating **more than just total testosterone**, doctors can determine whether **Low-T is caused by poor production, excessive binding, or excess conversion to estrogen**. This allows for a more **targeted and effective treatment approach**.

Timing Matters: When to Get Tested

Testosterone levels fluctuate throughout the day, with **peak production occurring in the early morning**. For the most accurate results, blood work should be done **between 7:00 and 10:00 AM**. Testing later in the day may show artificially low results, leading to **misdiagnosis or unnecessary concern**.

In some cases, a **second test on a different day** may be needed to confirm consistent low levels before making a diagnosis. Hormone levels can vary due to **sleep, diet, stress, and illness**, so a single test may not always provide a complete picture.

What to Do If Your Doctor Dismisses Your Symptoms

Many men experience symptoms of Low-T but are told their **testosterone levels are "normal"** because they fall within the standard reference range. However, this range is **broad**—typically from **250 to 1,000 ng/dL**—and what is "normal" on paper may not be optimal for an individual's health.

If symptoms persist despite being told that levels are "fine," it's important to:

- Request a **full hormone panel**, not just total testosterone.
- Look at **free testosterone levels**, which may be low even if total testosterone appears normal.
- Consider seeking a **second opinion from a doctor who specializes in hormone health**.

Proper testing is the foundation for **understanding and addressing Low-T effectively**. Without it, many men are left **struggling with symptoms without a clear answer**. Getting tested the right way ensures that the next steps—whether natural or medical—are based on **real, measurable data**, allowing for **better long-term results and a plan that works**.

Why Many Men Go Undiagnosed

Despite the clear impact low testosterone can have on energy, mood, body composition, and overall health, **many men never receive a proper diagnosis**. Some assume their symptoms are simply part of aging, while others seek medical help but **are dismissed by doctors who don't take hormonal health seriously**. The result? **Millions of men struggling with Low-T without knowing the real cause.**

One of the biggest barriers to diagnosis is that **the symptoms of Low-T often overlap with other conditions**. Fatigue, brain fog, depression, and weight gain can be mistakenly attributed to stress, poor sleep, or an unhealthy lifestyle. While these factors **can contribute to hormone imbalance**, they don't tell the full story—yet many doctors focus on these surface-level explanations rather than checking testosterone levels.

Another reason many men go undiagnosed is the **flawed approach to testosterone testing**. Since the "normal" range for testosterone is **incredibly broad**, men with symptoms are often told their levels are "fine" even when they are on the lower end of the spectrum. What's considered "normal" on a lab report may still be too low for a specific individual to **feel strong, energized, and mentally sharp**.

Common Misconceptions That Prevent Diagnosis

There are several myths surrounding Low-T that lead to **misdiagnosis or a failure to seek treatment**. Some of the most common include:

- **"Low testosterone only affects older men."** While testosterone does naturally decline with age, **younger men are increasingly being diagnosed with Low-T** due to lifestyle, diet, and environmental factors. Men in their 30s and 40s—sometimes even their 20s—can experience symptoms.

- **"If you work out and eat well, you can't have Low-T."** While **exercise and diet do play a major role in testosterone production**, they don't override other factors like genetics, stress, chemical exposure, or underlying medical conditions. Some men with great habits still experience a decline in testosterone due to **metabolic disorders, chronic inflammation, or excessive endurance training**.

- **"You don't need to test testosterone unless you have severe symptoms."** Many men assume that unless they have **zero energy, no sex drive, or severe depression**, their testosterone levels must be fine. But symptoms develop **gradually**, and catching Low-T early can **prevent further decline and long-term health risks**.

How to Advocate for Proper Testing

If a doctor dismisses concerns about Low-T, it's important to **push for the right tests or seek a second opinion**. Many men are told their symptoms are due to stress, aging, or lifestyle choices, when in reality, they have **a correctable hormone imbalance**.

When speaking to a doctor, key points to emphasize include:

- **Describing symptoms in detail**, including how they affect daily life and long-term health.
- **Asking for a complete hormone panel**, not just total testosterone.
- **Requesting a copy of lab results** to personally review levels and determine whether they are optimal, not just within range.
- **Bringing research or case studies** on the importance of free testosterone and SHBG levels in symptom assessment.

For men who suspect Low-T but have been ignored or misdiagnosed, **finding a doctor who specializes in hormone health** can be a game-changer. Many primary care doctors lack experience in **male hormone optimization**, but specialists in **endocrinology, urology, and men's health clinics** are often better equipped to properly evaluate and treat testosterone deficiencies.

The biggest mistake men make is **waiting too long to address Low-T**. Ignoring the symptoms doesn't make them go away—it allows them to **progress and worsen over time**. By recognizing the early warning signs and pushing for proper testing, men can take control of their hormonal health before **it impacts their long-term well-being and quality of life**.

When Should You Seek Treatment?

Many men experience symptoms of Low-T for years before taking action, often assuming that fatigue, mood swings, and weight gain are just part of getting older. While some decline in testosterone is natural, **there is a big difference between normal aging and clinically low testosterone**. The key question is: **At what point does Low-T require treatment?**

The answer depends on **both symptoms and lab results**. Some men with borderline testosterone levels feel perfectly fine, while others with slightly higher numbers experience severe fatigue, depression, and loss of motivation. That's why **symptoms matter just as much as test results**. If Low-T is interfering with energy, confidence, focus, or quality of life, it's worth addressing—whether through lifestyle changes, supplements, or medical treatment.

A good rule of thumb is: **If symptoms are persistent, getting worse, or affecting daily performance, it's time to take action.**

Mild, Moderate, and Severe Testosterone Deficiency

Low-T doesn't happen overnight. For many men, symptoms start slowly and **become more noticeable over time**. Recognizing where testosterone levels stand can help determine **the best approach for treatment**.

- **Mild Low-T** – Symptoms may include occasional fatigue, lower motivation, reduced stamina, or mild brain fog. Men in this stage can often **restore optimal levels through diet, exercise, stress management, and key supplements.**

- **Moderate Low-T** – Energy levels decline more noticeably, workouts become less effective, and libido drops. Mental fog increases, and **mood swings or irritability become more common**. At this stage, lifestyle changes are still helpful, but **medical options may also be worth considering.**

- **Severe Low-T** – Symptoms now significantly impact **quality of life**. Fatigue is overwhelming, depression and anxiety worsen, muscle loss accelerates, and sexual function declines sharply. **At this stage, testosterone replacement therapy (TRT) or other hormone-supporting medications may be necessary.**

Understanding where testosterone levels fall **helps determine the best treatment strategy**. The sooner Low-T is addressed, the easier it is to restore **energy, strength, and motivation before symptoms become more difficult to reverse.**

Why Treating Low-T Early Matters

Some men hesitate to seek treatment, assuming they can just **power through** symptoms or wait for things to improve on their own. However, ignoring Low-T **only allows the problem to worsen**.

Left untreated, Low-T can lead to:

- **Increased risk of obesity and diabetes** due to poor metabolism.
- **Weakened bones and muscles**, leading to a greater risk of injury.
- **Heart health issues**, including higher blood pressure and cholesterol levels.
- **Cognitive decline**, making it harder to concentrate and retain information.
- **Chronic fatigue and emotional instability**, reducing quality of life.

The good news is that **Low-T is one of the most manageable conditions** when addressed early. Whether through natural methods or medical intervention, testosterone levels **can be restored, allowing men to feel sharper, stronger, and more like themselves again**. The most important step is recognizing **when it's time to take action**—because the longer Low-T is ignored, the more impact it has on long-term health.

Chapter 3: Why Testosterone Levels Decline – Causes and Risk Factors

Age-Related Testosterone Decline – What's Normal?

Testosterone naturally declines with age, but the rate at which this happens—and how much of an impact it has—varies widely between individuals. In a **healthy aging process**, testosterone decreases **gradually**, at about **1% per year after the age of 30**. This slow decline doesn't always lead to noticeable symptoms, especially for men who maintain good health and strong metabolic function.

However, for some men, testosterone **drops faster than expected**, leading to the early onset of Low-T symptoms. By the time they reach their **40s or 50s**, they may experience significant **loss of energy, muscle mass, libido, and cognitive sharpness**—far beyond what would be considered normal aging.

Aging alone doesn't automatically cause severe Low-T, but it **increases the likelihood**

of hormonal imbalance when combined with other factors like:

- **Chronic stress and elevated cortisol levels**.
- **Poor sleep quality and lack of recovery time**.
- **Excess body fat and insulin resistance**.
- **Reduced physical activity and loss of muscle mass**.

Many men in their 30s and 40s today are seeing **testosterone levels that previous generations didn't experience until their 60s**. This raises an important question: **Is testosterone decline truly a part of aging, or is it a result of modern lifestyle factors accelerating the process?**

The Difference Between Healthy Aging and Clinical Low-T

Some level of testosterone decline is expected, but not **every man develops symptoms of Low-T**. The key difference is how well the body **adapts** to these hormonal changes. A man who maintains **good muscle mass, a healthy metabolism, and stable**

hormone function may still experience a decrease in testosterone over time but **won't necessarily feel the negative effects**.

In contrast, men with **poor metabolic health, chronic stress, or excessive weight gain** are more likely to see a **rapid and noticeable drop in testosterone**. This leads to:

- A sharp decline in **energy, strength, and libido**.
- Increased **belly fat and loss of muscle tone**.
- Difficulty concentrating, mood swings, and emotional instability.

The key takeaway is this: **Aging doesn't have to mean losing testosterone at an unhealthy rate**. While some decline is natural, much of what is considered "normal aging" is actually **preventable**—and even reversible—with the right approach.

Testosterone decline can be **slowed, minimized, and in some cases reversed** through lifestyle strategies, nutrition, and targeted medical treatments. Recognizing **when testosterone is declining too quickly** allows men to take control before symptoms worsen, ensuring they maintain **vitality, confidence, and strength well into later years**.

The Role of Lifestyle in Low Testosterone

While testosterone naturally declines with age, lifestyle plays a major role in **how quickly and how severely** it drops. Many modern habits **disrupt hormone production**, leading to an acceleration of Low-T symptoms that could otherwise be prevented. The way a man **eats, sleeps, moves, and handles stress** all contribute to his body's ability to maintain **healthy testosterone levels**.

One of the biggest testosterone killers is **chronic stress**. When the body is constantly under pressure, it produces **high levels of cortisol**, the primary stress hormone. Cortisol and testosterone have an **inverse relationship**—when cortisol rises, testosterone drops. This is because the body prioritizes survival over reproduction, shifting resources away from testosterone production.

Men who experience **constant work stress, poor sleep, or emotional strain** often see their **testosterone levels decline faster** than those with better stress management. Over time, this can lead to **fatigue, mental fog, irritability, and lower drive**, both physically and mentally.

The Impact of Diet, Alcohol, and Inactivity

What a man eats directly affects his **hormonal health**, and poor diet choices are a major contributor to **Low-T in modern men**. Diets high in **processed foods, refined carbohydrates, and excessive sugar** lead to **insulin resistance, weight gain, and inflammation**—all of which disrupt testosterone production. The body **needs healthy fats, proteins, and key nutrients** to synthesize testosterone effectively.

Inactivity is another major factor. **Testosterone responds to physical demand**—if the body doesn't need strength, endurance, or muscle, testosterone production slows down. Men who spend long hours sitting and **don't engage in regular strength**

training often experience a decline in testosterone **much earlier** than those who stay physically active.

Alcohol also plays a significant role in **lowering testosterone levels**. Regular consumption, especially of **beer and hard liquor**, raises estrogen levels, increases cortisol, and damages liver function—all of which reduce testosterone production. **Excessive drinking over time leads to hormonal imbalances that make it harder for the body to regulate testosterone naturally**.

How Lifestyle Choices Can Preserve or Destroy Testosterone

The good news is that **lifestyle-related testosterone decline is reversible**. Men who focus on **reducing stress, eating nutrient-dense foods, prioritizing sleep, and engaging in the right types of exercise** can often restore **optimal testosterone levels without medical intervention**.

However, ignoring these factors allows testosterone to decline **much faster than necessary**, leading to **fatigue, weight gain, mood instability, and loss of confidence**. Many men accept these changes as part of getting older, but in reality, they are **the result of habits that can be adjusted**.

Recognizing the connection between **daily choices and hormone balance** is one of the most powerful tools for preventing Low-T. The body is constantly responding to **how it is treated**, and by making the right changes, testosterone levels can often be **preserved, stabilized, and even increased naturally**.

Environmental Factors That Lower Testosterone

Modern living comes with an **unexpected threat to male hormone health**—environmental toxins. Every day, men are exposed to chemicals that **disrupt endocrine function**, interfering with the body's natural ability to produce and regulate testosterone. These substances, known as **endocrine**

disruptors, are found in **plastics, pesticides, personal care products, and even household cleaning supplies**.

One of the most common and harmful endocrine disruptors is **bisphenol A (BPA)**, a chemical found in **plastic bottles, food containers, and canned goods**. BPA mimics estrogen in the body, leading to **hormonal imbalances that suppress testosterone production**. Studies have shown that **men with high BPA exposure tend to have lower free testosterone levels**, along with increased body fat and insulin resistance.

Another major culprit is **phthalates**, chemicals used in **cosmetics, deodorants, shampoos, and scented products**. Phthalates interfere with the body's ability to produce testosterone by disrupting signals from the brain to the testes. **Regular exposure can lead to reduced sperm quality, lower libido, and an increased risk of Low-T over time**.

The Hidden Dangers of Processed Foods and Chemical Exposure

Beyond personal care products, **the modern diet is loaded with hormone-disrupting substances**. Many processed foods contain **preservatives, artificial flavorings, and chemical additives** that negatively affect testosterone levels. Additionally, foods sprayed with pesticides contain **residues that can mimic estrogen in the body**, further throwing off hormonal balance.

Men who consume high amounts of **processed meats, fast food, and heavily packaged products** are unknowingly exposing themselves to a **constant stream of hormone-disrupting chemicals**. These substances accumulate in the body, leading to **higher estrogen levels, increased fat storage, and suppressed testosterone production**.

Other environmental factors that contribute to Low-T include:

- **Heavy metal exposure** – Lead and mercury, often found in contaminated water and seafood, have been linked to testosterone suppression.

- **Air pollution** – Persistent exposure to **toxins in the air** can increase inflammation and negatively affect hormone regulation.
- **Nonstick cookware** – Chemicals used in **Teflon coatings** have been shown to lower sperm quality and interfere with testosterone production.

How to Reduce Environmental Testosterone Disruptors

Avoiding all environmental toxins is impossible, but **limiting exposure** can make a significant difference. Some of the most effective ways to reduce endocrine disruptors include:

- **Using glass or stainless steel containers** instead of plastic for food and drinks.
- **Switching to natural grooming products** that are free from parabens and phthalates.
- **Eating organic whenever possible** to avoid pesticide-heavy produce.
- **Filtering tap water** to remove heavy metals and chemicals.

- **Choosing cookware made from cast iron, stainless steel, or ceramic** instead of nonstick coatings.

While these changes may seem small, **they add up over time**, allowing the body to regulate testosterone levels more efficiently. By reducing exposure to harmful chemicals and prioritizing a cleaner environment, men can **support healthy hormone production and protect long-term vitality**.

The Link Between Obesity, Insulin Resistance, and Low-T

One of the most overlooked causes of Low-T is **excess body fat**, particularly around the **abdomen and chest**. While testosterone is often thought of as a hormone that influences body composition, the relationship goes both ways—**excess fat can directly lower testosterone levels**, creating a cycle that is difficult to break.

Fat cells, especially those in the belly, contain an enzyme called **aromatase**, which converts testosterone into estrogen. This means that the more body fat a man carries, the more testosterone is lost to estrogen conversion. Over time, this leads to a **hormonal imbalance where estrogen levels rise while testosterone levels decline**, causing symptoms such as:

- Increased **belly fat and difficulty losing weight**.
- Loss of **muscle mass and strength**.
- **Mood swings and emotional instability** due to hormonal shifts.
- **Lower libido and sexual function issues**.

In addition to increasing estrogen, excess fat **worsens insulin resistance**, a condition where the body struggles to regulate blood sugar properly. When insulin resistance develops, the body produces more insulin, which **further suppresses testosterone production**. This is why men with **obesity and metabolic disorders** are far more likely to suffer from Low-T than those with a leaner body composition.

How Metabolic Health Influences Testosterone

Testosterone and **metabolic health** are closely linked. A strong metabolism **supports testosterone production**, while metabolic dysfunction suppresses it. When insulin resistance develops, the body experiences:

- **Chronic inflammation**, which interferes with hormone signaling.
- **Higher cortisol levels**, leading to further testosterone suppression.
- **Lower energy and increased fatigue**, making it harder to stay active and maintain a healthy weight.

Men with **pre-diabetes, type 2 diabetes, or excessive visceral fat** often find themselves in a downward spiral where **weight gain lowers testosterone, and lower testosterone makes it harder to lose weight**. This is why addressing metabolic health is one of the most **effective natural ways to restore testosterone levels**.

Breaking the Cycle: Restoring Testosterone Through Fat Loss

The good news is that testosterone levels often **improve significantly** when men reduce body fat and improve insulin sensitivity. Studies have shown that:

- Losing just **5–10% of body fat** can result in a **natural increase in testosterone production**.
- Strength training and **high-intensity interval training (HIIT)** help lower insulin resistance while stimulating testosterone release.
- A diet focused on **whole, nutrient-dense foods** reduces inflammation and stabilizes blood sugar, making it easier for the body to produce testosterone.

By improving metabolic health, men can **reverse the hormonal imbalances that contribute to Low-T**, leading to better energy, improved strength, and restored confidence. **Addressing body fat isn't just about aesthetics—it's a key step toward long-term testosterone optimization and overall well-being.**

Medical Conditions That Lower Testosterone

While lifestyle and environmental factors play a major role in testosterone decline, **certain medical conditions can directly disrupt hormone production and regulation**. Some conditions affect the testes, preventing them from producing enough testosterone, while others interfere with **the brain's ability to signal testosterone production properly**. Identifying these underlying medical causes is crucial, as they often require **a different approach than lifestyle adjustments alone**.

One of the most common medical causes of Low-T is **hypogonadism**, a condition where the testes fail to produce enough testosterone. Hypogonadism can be **primary** (caused by testicular damage or dysfunction) or **secondary** (caused by issues in the brain's hormone-regulating centers, such as the pituitary gland or hypothalamus).

Men with primary hypogonadism may have experienced:

- **Testicular injuries** from trauma, surgery, or infections like mumps.

- **Radiation or chemotherapy treatments**, which can damage testosterone-producing cells.
- **Genetic conditions**, such as Klinefelter syndrome, that impair testosterone production.

Secondary hypogonadism is often linked to **hormonal signaling problems**, where the brain does not send enough luteinizing hormone (LH) and follicle-stimulating hormone (FSH) to stimulate testosterone production. This can be caused by:

- **Pituitary gland disorders** (tumors, inflammation, or hormonal imbalances).
- **Chronic stress or excessive cortisol levels**, which suppress testosterone regulation.
- **Obesity and insulin resistance**, which interfere with brain-to-testes communication.

Why Chronic Illnesses Affect Testosterone Levels

Many chronic diseases have a **direct impact on testosterone production**, either by increasing inflammation, disrupting hormone balance, or causing damage to testosterone-producing tissues. Some of the most common include:

- **Diabetes** – High blood sugar and insulin resistance reduce the body's ability to produce and regulate testosterone. Men with type 2 diabetes have significantly higher rates of Low-T.
- **Thyroid disorders** – Both hypothyroidism and hyperthyroidism can alter testosterone levels and lead to hormonal imbalances.
- **Chronic inflammation conditions** – Diseases like rheumatoid arthritis and inflammatory bowel disease raise cortisol levels, which suppress testosterone production.
- **Kidney and liver disease** – These organs help metabolize and regulate hormones, so dysfunction can contribute to testosterone imbalances.

The Impact of Medications on Testosterone

Some commonly prescribed medications can also contribute to Low-T, either by interfering with testosterone production or increasing estrogen levels. These include:

- **Opioids and pain medications**, which suppress hormone signaling from the brain.
- **Antidepressants and anti-anxiety medications**, which can lower libido and testosterone levels over time.
- **Statins and cholesterol-lowering drugs**, which may reduce testosterone by affecting cholesterol, a key building block for hormone production.
- **Corticosteroids**, such as prednisone, which elevate cortisol and suppress testosterone.

When to Consider Medical Testing for Low-T

For men who suspect that **an underlying medical condition is contributing to their testosterone decline**, it's important to undergo **comprehensive hormone testing**. This includes checking:

- **Total and free testosterone levels**.
- **LH and FSH**, to determine if the problem is with the brain or the testes.
- **Prolactin levels**, which can indicate pituitary dysfunction.
- **Thyroid function**, to rule out thyroid-related hormone imbalances.

While lifestyle changes can help **many men restore optimal testosterone levels**, those with underlying medical conditions may require **more specialized treatments**. Understanding these potential medical causes ensures that men can **address Low-T effectively and improve overall health** rather than just treating the symptoms.

Can Low-T Be Prevented?

While testosterone naturally declines with age, many of the **factors that accelerate Low-T are within a man's control**. By making **smart lifestyle choices early**, it's possible to **slow, minimize, or even prevent** testosterone decline. The key is focusing on habits that **support natural testosterone**

production, while avoiding the common pitfalls that lead to hormonal imbalance.

One of the most powerful tools for preventing Low-T is **maintaining a healthy body composition**. Since **excess fat—especially around the abdomen—converts testosterone into estrogen**, staying lean helps preserve **hormonal balance and overall metabolic health**. Regular strength training and physical activity keep **testosterone levels stable**, ensuring that the body continues to produce and regulate hormones efficiently.

The Impact of Exercise, Diet, and Stress Management

Testosterone thrives when the body is **active, well-nourished, and properly rested**. Men who follow these foundational habits are far less likely to experience **early or severe testosterone decline**:

- **Strength training** stimulates natural testosterone production by increasing muscle demand. Compound exercises

like squats, deadlifts, and bench presses are especially effective.
- **A diet rich in healthy fats, protein, and key micronutrients** provides the building blocks for testosterone synthesis. Nutrients like **zinc, magnesium, vitamin D, and omega-3s** play a direct role in hormone regulation.
- **Stress reduction techniques**, such as meditation, breathing exercises, and relaxation strategies, help lower **cortisol levels**, preventing testosterone suppression. Chronic stress is one of the biggest contributors to hormonal imbalance.
- **Consistent, high-quality sleep** is essential. The majority of testosterone production happens during deep sleep, and even **one week of sleep deprivation can lower testosterone levels** by as much as 15%.

Avoiding Testosterone-Killing Habits

Just as certain habits support testosterone, others can **accelerate its decline**. The most damaging include:

- **Sedentary lifestyles** – Long periods of inactivity signal to the body that **testosterone production is not a priority**.
- **Excessive alcohol consumption** – Alcohol increases estrogen levels and damages the liver's ability to **process hormones efficiently**.
- **Endocrine-disrupting chemicals** – Avoiding **plastics, processed foods, and artificial fragrances** helps limit exposure to hormone-disrupting toxins.
- **Chronic sleep deprivation** – Poor sleep quality directly lowers testosterone and **raises cortisol**, making hormonal recovery difficult.

Taking a Long-Term Approach to Testosterone Health

Testosterone management isn't just about **fixing a problem once symptoms appear**—it's about **long-term optimization**. By building **consistent, sustainable habits**, men can maintain **higher testosterone levels naturally**, preserving their **energy, strength, and mental sharpness for decades**.

The earlier these habits are developed, the easier it is to **prevent Low-T from becoming an issue**. Even for men already experiencing symptoms, making these changes can lead to **significant improvements**, sometimes restoring testosterone levels without the need for medical intervention.

By taking control of **diet, exercise, stress, and sleep**, men can **support their testosterone production naturally**, ensuring that they continue to feel strong, motivated, and vital—no matter their age.

Chapter 4: Natural Ways to Boost Testosterone – Lifestyle, Diet, and Exercise

The Best Foods for Naturally Increasing Testosterone

What a man eats has a **direct impact on testosterone production**. The body relies on specific nutrients to synthesize hormones, and a diet lacking in these essentials can **lead to hormonal imbalances, sluggish metabolism, and a gradual decline in testosterone levels**. The good news? **Certain foods are proven to support healthy testosterone production**, helping to optimize levels naturally.

One of the most important nutrients for testosterone is **zinc**, a mineral that plays a vital role in hormone regulation. Studies show that **men with low zinc intake often have lower testosterone levels**, while supplementing with zinc can help **restore and maintain optimal hormone function**. Foods rich in zinc include:

- Oysters – One of the highest natural sources of zinc.
- Grass-fed beef – Provides zinc, iron, and high-quality protein.
- Pumpkin seeds – A plant-based option packed with zinc and magnesium.

Another essential nutrient is **vitamin D**, which acts as a **natural testosterone booster**. Research has found that men with sufficient vitamin D levels **tend to have higher testosterone** than those who are deficient. The best dietary sources include:

- Fatty fish like salmon, mackerel, and sardines.
- Egg yolks, which also contain cholesterol, a building block for testosterone.
- Fortified dairy products, though sunshine exposure remains the best source of vitamin D.

The Role of Healthy Fats in Testosterone Production

For years, dietary fat was demonized, but **healthy fats are crucial for testosterone synthesis**. Testosterone is derived from cholesterol, so a **diet too low in fat can actually lower testosterone production**. The key is focusing on **the right types of fats**:

- **Saturated fats** (in moderation) from sources like grass-fed beef, butter, and coconut oil.
- **Monounsaturated fats** from olive oil, avocados, and nuts.
- **Omega-3 fatty acids**, which reduce inflammation and support hormonal balance, found in salmon, walnuts, and flaxseeds.

Carbohydrates also play a role in **testosterone and energy regulation**. While low-carb diets can be beneficial for weight loss, **going too low in carbs for too long may lead to cortisol spikes**, which can suppress testosterone. The best approach is to consume **complex, unprocessed carbs**, such as:

- Sweet potatoes and other root vegetables.
- Whole grains like quinoa and oats.

- Dark leafy greens, which also provide magnesium—another essential testosterone-supporting mineral.

What to Avoid: Foods That Lower Testosterone

Just as some foods **enhance testosterone production**, others **work against it**, leading to hormonal imbalances and lower levels. The biggest offenders include:

- **Processed foods high in trans fats**, which increase inflammation and disrupt hormone function.
- **Excess sugar and refined carbs**, which lead to insulin resistance, a known testosterone suppressor.
- **Soy-based products**, which contain phytoestrogens that mimic estrogen in the body, potentially interfering with testosterone production.
- **Alcohol, especially beer**, which increases estrogen and disrupts liver function, making it harder for the body to regulate hormones.

By making simple but **effective dietary changes**, men can **naturally support testosterone levels, enhance overall health, and improve energy, strength, and mental clarity**—all without the need for drastic interventions. The right foods serve as **the foundation for long-term hormone balance and vitality**.

How Strength Training and Exercise Improve Testosterone

Testosterone is a hormone that thrives on **physical demand**. When the body is challenged through **resistance training and high-intensity exercise**, testosterone production increases naturally. This is why strength training is one of the most **effective natural methods for boosting and maintaining optimal testosterone levels**.

Lifting weights signals the body that **muscle needs to be built and preserved**, which in turn triggers a rise in **testosterone and growth hormone production**. The best types of workouts for supporting testosterone include:

- **Compound exercises** – Movements like squats, deadlifts, bench presses, and pull-ups engage multiple muscle groups, leading to **higher testosterone release**.
- **Heavy lifting with lower reps** – Working in the **4-8 rep range with heavier resistance** has been shown to stimulate greater testosterone production compared to high-rep endurance training.
- **High-intensity interval training (HIIT)** – Short bursts of intense activity, followed by brief rest periods, can **increase testosterone and growth hormone levels while burning fat**.

Men who train consistently experience **higher baseline testosterone levels**, better metabolic health, and improved body composition. However, there's a balance—**too much cardio or endurance training can actually lower testosterone levels** if recovery isn't prioritized.

The Downside of Overtraining

While regular exercise is essential for maintaining healthy testosterone, **overtraining without proper recovery can have the opposite effect**. Excessive training—especially long-duration cardio—**raises cortisol levels**, the body's primary stress hormone. Since cortisol and testosterone work in opposition, **elevated cortisol can suppress testosterone production**.

Men who engage in **long-distance running, extreme endurance training, or excessive daily workouts** without enough rest may experience:

- **Increased fatigue and slower recovery times.**
- **Muscle loss rather than growth.**
- **Higher stress and lower motivation over time.**

The key is **balance**. Combining **strength training, short bursts of high-intensity cardio, and proper recovery** provides the best results for maintaining testosterone naturally.

Optimizing Recovery for Testosterone Production

Muscles and hormones don't just grow in the gym—they **develop and regulate during recovery**. Prioritizing rest is just as important as working out when it comes to keeping testosterone levels high. Some of the most effective recovery strategies include:

- **Prioritizing sleep** – Testosterone is produced primarily during deep sleep. **Men who get less than 6 hours per night often see a significant drop in testosterone levels**.
- **Rest days between intense workouts** – Lifting heavy every single day without recovery can spike cortisol and reduce testosterone.
- **Eating enough calories and protein** – Undereating, especially in protein and healthy fats, can lower testosterone production.

By **training smart, lifting heavy, and giving the body time to recover**, men can naturally boost their **testosterone levels, increase muscle mass, and maintain long-term vitality**. Strength training isn't just about looking good—it's one of the most powerful ways to **support hormone health and keep testosterone levels optimized for life**.

Why Sleep Is Critical for Hormone Balance

Testosterone production is directly tied to **the quality and duration of sleep**. In fact, the majority of testosterone release happens **during deep sleep cycles**, particularly in the **early morning hours** when levels peak. This is why **poor sleep is one of the fastest ways to lower testosterone**, leading to **chronic fatigue, reduced motivation, and sluggish recovery from workouts**.

Studies have shown that **just one week of sleep deprivation can lower testosterone levels by up to 15%**. Men who consistently sleep **less than six hours per night** are at an even greater risk of developing **Low-T, increased cortisol, and metabolic dysfunction**.

The relationship between sleep and testosterone works both ways—**low testosterone can also make sleep worse**. Many men with Low-T experience:

- **Difficulty falling or staying asleep.**
- **More frequent nighttime awakenings.**
- **Daytime fatigue, even after a full night of rest.**

This creates a cycle where **poor sleep lowers testosterone, and low testosterone makes sleep quality worse**, leading to a gradual decline in **physical and mental performance**.

How to Optimize Sleep for Maximum Testosterone Production

Improving sleep is one of the **simplest and most effective ways to boost testosterone naturally**. The goal is to **increase deep, restorative sleep**, which allows the body to release the most testosterone. Some key strategies include:

- **Getting 7–9 hours of sleep per night** – Men who sleep at least 7 hours typically have **higher baseline testosterone levels** than those who sleep less.
- **Going to bed at the same time every night** – A consistent sleep schedule **helps regulate the body's natural hormone cycles**.
- **Eliminating blue light exposure before bed** – Screens from phones, tablets, and TVs **suppress melatonin**, the hormone that signals the body to sleep.
- **Lowering bedroom temperature** – The body sleeps best at a **cooler temperature (around 65–68°F or 18–20°C)**, which promotes deeper sleep.
- **Avoiding alcohol and heavy meals before bedtime** – Both disrupt deep sleep and interfere with **testosterone release overnight**.

Incorporating these simple changes **can significantly improve testosterone levels, energy, and overall health**. Many men notice **better mood, sharper focus, and improved workouts** just by prioritizing high-quality sleep.

Since **testosterone and sleep are so closely connected**, ensuring **restorative sleep** is one of the **most powerful natural strategies** for maintaining long-term hormonal balance.

Stress Management and Cortisol Reduction

Testosterone and cortisol—the body's primary stress hormone—have an **inverse relationship**. When cortisol levels rise due to **chronic stress, anxiety, or overwork**, testosterone levels **drop**. This is because the body prioritizes **survival over reproduction**, shifting resources away from hormone production that isn't immediately necessary for dealing with stress.

In today's fast-paced world, **constant exposure to stressors**—whether from work, finances, relationships, or lack of rest—can keep cortisol levels **chronically elevated**, leading to:

- **Fatigue and burnout** even after a full night's sleep.
- **Difficulty building muscle and increased fat storage**, especially around the belly.
- **Irritability, mood swings, and lack of motivation**.
- **Low libido and reduced drive in all areas of life**.

While short-term stress is normal and even beneficial in some situations, **chronic stress disrupts hormonal balance** and **accelerates testosterone decline**. The good news is that by managing stress effectively, men can **naturally support testosterone production** and regain a sense of energy and control.

Practical Ways to Reduce Stress and Support Testosterone

Lowering cortisol and maintaining balanced testosterone levels requires **active stress management techniques**. Some of the most effective strategies include:

- **Meditation and deep breathing exercises** – Just 5–10 minutes a day of mindful breathing can **lower cortisol and improve mental clarity**.
- **Cold exposure and contrast showers** – Exposure to cold water has been shown to **reduce stress hormones and stimulate testosterone production**.
- **Regular physical activity** – Exercise not only boosts testosterone but also **helps clear excess cortisol from the bloodstream**, reducing stress naturally.
- **Sunlight and nature exposure** – Spending time outdoors, especially in natural settings, has been proven to **lower stress hormones and improve mood**.
- **Limiting screen time and digital overload** – Constant exposure to emails, news, and notifications can **keep the brain in a heightened stress state**, making it harder for testosterone to stay balanced.

Men who make **stress management a daily habit** often notice:

- **Better mood stability and resilience**.
- **Improved focus and mental sharpness**.

- **Easier fat loss and muscle maintenance**.
- **Higher libido and overall motivation**.

Since **testosterone thrives in a low-stress environment**, keeping cortisol in check is a critical part of **any natural hormone optimization plan**. Making **small, daily adjustments** to lower stress can have a **massive impact** on energy, confidence, and long-term testosterone health.

Which Supplements Actually Work?

While lifestyle changes like **exercise, sleep, and stress management** are the foundation for healthy testosterone levels, **certain supplements can provide additional support**. The key is knowing which ones are **scientifically backed** and which are just marketing hype. Many so-called "testosterone boosters" fail to deliver real results, but **a few specific nutrients have been shown to support hormone production and balance**.

Proven Supplements for Testosterone Support

- **Vitamin D3** – Often called the "sunshine vitamin," vitamin D plays a crucial role in **testosterone production and overall hormone balance**. Studies show that men with higher vitamin D levels **tend to have higher testosterone**, while deficiency is linked to **Low-T, fatigue, and poor immune function**. If getting enough sun exposure isn't possible, supplementing with **3,000–5,000 IU per day** can be beneficial.

- **Zinc** – An essential mineral for **testosterone synthesis, immune function, and sperm production**. Even mild zinc deficiency can lead to **lower testosterone and reduced libido**. Foods like oysters, beef, and pumpkin seeds provide zinc, but supplementation (15–30 mg per day) can help those not getting enough from diet.

- **Magnesium** – Supports **free testosterone levels** by reducing the binding effects of **sex hormone-binding globulin (SHBG)**, which can make testosterone more available in the body. Magnesium also improves **sleep and recovery**, two factors crucial for maintaining optimal testosterone.

- **Ashwagandha** – An adaptogenic herb that **reduces cortisol (stress hormone) and supports testosterone levels**. Several studies have shown that ashwagandha supplementation can **increase testosterone by 10–20% while improving stress resilience**.

- **DHEA (Dehydroepiandrosterone)** – A precursor hormone that **helps the body produce more testosterone naturally**. Some studies suggest it can be beneficial for older men or those with naturally declining levels, but it should be used cautiously and under medical supervision.

What About Herbal Testosterone Boosters?

Many testosterone booster supplements on the market include **herbs like tribulus**

terrestris, fenugreek, and tongkat ali. While these may have some mild libido-enhancing effects, **they don't significantly raise testosterone in men with normal levels**. However, some men report improvements in **energy and mood** with certain herbal extracts, so they may be worth experimenting with.

What to Avoid: Supplements That Don't Work

- **Over-the-counter testosterone boosters** – Most are underdosed or contain ingredients with **no real impact on testosterone production**.
- **Excessive soy-based supplements** – Some plant estrogens, like those found in soy protein powders, may **increase estrogen levels** and interfere with testosterone.
- **Prohormones and unregulated substances** – Some "testosterone boosters" contain **hormonal precursors** that can disrupt natural testosterone production rather than support it.

The Best Strategy: A Combination Approach

No supplement alone will dramatically increase testosterone—**but when combined with proper diet, sleep, exercise, and stress reduction**, these nutrients **can help optimize testosterone naturally**. Instead of chasing quick fixes, the most effective approach is to **focus on long-term hormone health**, using supplements as a tool rather than a crutch.

By choosing **science-backed supplements and pairing them with lifestyle improvements**, men can experience **better energy, improved performance, and long-term hormonal stability** without relying on synthetic treatments.

Testosterone-Killing Habits to Avoid

While many factors contribute to **healthy testosterone production**, certain habits can **drastically lower testosterone levels**, often without men realizing it. Modern lifestyles are filled with hidden testosterone disruptors, and even small daily habits can **chip away at hormone balance over time**. Avoiding these common mistakes is just as important as taking the right steps to **boost testosterone naturally**.

1. Chronic Sleep Deprivation

Testosterone production **peaks during deep sleep**, and men who regularly sleep fewer than six hours a night can experience **a significant drop in testosterone levels**. Poor sleep disrupts the body's **natural hormone rhythms**, leading to:

- Increased **cortisol** (stress hormone), which suppresses testosterone.
- Reduced **growth hormone release**, which supports muscle and recovery.
- Lower **energy, libido, and motivation**, making everything feel more difficult.

Prioritizing **7–9 hours of high-quality sleep** is one of the most effective ways to **naturally restore testosterone** and improve overall health.

2. Excessive Alcohol Consumption

While occasional alcohol intake is fine, **regular or excessive drinking can lower testosterone levels**—especially beer, which contains phytoestrogens that **increase estrogen levels in men**. Alcohol also:

- Increases **cortisol production**, further suppressing testosterone.
- Disrupts **liver function**, reducing the body's ability to **metabolize and regulate hormones**.
- Lowers **sleep quality**, compounding the negative effects on testosterone.

Men looking to optimize their testosterone should **limit alcohol intake**, especially **beer and high-sugar mixed drinks**.

3. High Stress and Constant Cortisol Spikes

Chronic stress is one of the **biggest testosterone killers**. When cortisol remains elevated for long periods, **testosterone production slows down**. This is why men who are constantly **overworked, anxious, or overwhelmed** often feel exhausted and unmotivated.

Stress management techniques such as **meditation, deep breathing, cold exposure, and exercise** can help **lower cortisol and support natural testosterone production.**

4. A Diet High in Processed Foods and Sugar

Poor nutrition is a major driver of **Low-T and metabolic dysfunction**. Diets high in **refined sugars, seed oils, and processed foods** contribute to:

- **Insulin resistance**, which lowers testosterone.
- **Excess body fat**, leading to increased **estrogen conversion**.
- **Chronic inflammation**, which disrupts hormone balance.

Focusing on **whole, nutrient-dense foods**—including lean proteins, healthy fats, and fiber-rich carbohydrates—helps **support long-term testosterone production.**

5. Endocrine-Disrupting Chemicals (EDCs)

Modern environments are filled with **hormone-disrupting chemicals**, many of which mimic estrogen and **suppress testosterone**. Some of the worst offenders include:

- **Plastics (BPA and phthalates)** – Found in water bottles, food containers, and canned goods

Chapter 5: Medical Treatments for Low Testosterone – What Works and What to Avoid

When Is TRT Necessary?

Testosterone replacement therapy (TRT) is often seen as the **go-to solution for Low-T**, but it's not always the first or best option. Many men can **boost testosterone naturally through lifestyle changes, diet, exercise, and supplements**. However, in cases where testosterone is **severely low and symptoms are significantly impacting quality of life**, TRT may be necessary.

Doctors typically recommend TRT when:

- **Testosterone levels are consistently below 300 ng/dL** on multiple tests.
- Symptoms like **fatigue, low libido, depression, and muscle loss** are persistent despite lifestyle changes.
- Other hormone-related issues, such as **pituitary dysfunction**, prevent natural testosterone production.

- A man's body is no longer capable of producing adequate testosterone due to **age, injury, or medical conditions**.

While TRT can be life-changing for men with clinically low testosterone, **it's not a one-size-fits-all solution**. Some men benefit greatly, while others experience **side effects or complications that require careful monitoring**.

Who Should Think Twice About TRT?

Not every man with low testosterone needs TRT. Some cases of Low-T are **temporary or caused by fixable issues**, such as:

- **Chronic stress and high cortisol levels** suppressing testosterone production.
- **Poor sleep, diet, and lack of exercise** contributing to hormonal imbalance.
- **Vitamin and mineral deficiencies**, particularly in zinc, magnesium, and vitamin D.

For men whose testosterone is only slightly below optimal, **natural interventions should always be attempted first** before committing to long-term hormone therapy. Since TRT affects the body's natural production, **once a man starts, his body may become dependent on external testosterone**, making it difficult to come off therapy later.

The Key to Success with TRT

When used correctly, TRT can be **an effective way to restore energy, strength, and vitality**. However, the key is **individualized treatment**—dosages and delivery methods should be tailored to each person. This is why working with an **experienced doctor who specializes in hormone health** is crucial.

For men considering TRT, **understanding both the benefits and the potential downsides** ensures that the decision is made **with long-term health in mind**. Before starting, men should be aware of **alternative treatments**, the importance of ongoing monitoring, and how TRT may affect other aspects of their health, such as fertility and cardiovascular function.

The Different Forms of Testosterone Replacement Therapy

Once a man is diagnosed with **clinically low testosterone** and decides to pursue TRT, the next question is: **What's the best method of treatment?** There is no one-size-fits-all approach—different forms of TRT have varying levels of convenience, effectiveness, and potential side effects. The right choice depends on **lifestyle, personal preference, and how the body responds** to each delivery method.

1. Testosterone Injections

One of the most common and effective forms of TRT is **injectable testosterone**, typically administered as **testosterone cypionate or testosterone enanthate**. These injections are:

- Given **intramuscularly (IM) or subcutaneously** every 1–2 weeks, depending on dosage.
- Often **self-administered at home**, making them a convenient option for many men.

- Relatively **affordable compared to other TRT methods**.

The downside is that **testosterone levels fluctuate between doses**, sometimes leading to **mood swings, energy dips, or symptoms returning before the next shot**. To avoid this, some men prefer **smaller injections given more frequently**, such as every **3–4 days instead of weekly**.

2. Topical Testosterone Gels and Creams

Testosterone gels and creams offer a **non-invasive alternative** to injections. These are applied **daily to the skin**, usually on the arms, shoulders, or thighs, and allow testosterone to absorb **gradually into the bloodstream**.

Advantages:

- **No needles or injections required.**
- **More stable hormone levels** with daily application.

Disadvantages:

- **Risk of transferring testosterone to others** through skin contact.
- **Absorption rates vary**, meaning some men may not get consistent results.
- **More expensive over time** compared to injections.

3. Testosterone Patches

Transdermal patches release **a controlled dose of testosterone throughout the day**, avoiding some of the fluctuations seen with injections. However, they come with **skin irritation issues** for many men and can be **less effective if not properly absorbed**.

4. Testosterone Pellets (Subcutaneous Implants)

Pellets are small, slow-release implants **inserted under the skin**, typically in the **hip or buttock area**, where they **release testosterone gradually over 3–6 months**.

Advantages:

- **No need for daily or weekly dosing**—once implanted, they provide **long-term, steady testosterone levels**.
- **Fewer hormone fluctuations compared to injections**.

Disadvantages:

- **Requires a minor surgical procedure to insert and remove pellets**.
- **Dosing adjustments are difficult**—if levels are too high or too low, it takes months to correct.
- **Higher cost upfront** compared to injections.

5. Oral Testosterone (Less Common)

Oral testosterone is **not widely used** due to concerns about **liver toxicity and inconsistent absorption**. Newer formulations, such as **testosterone undecanoate**, are designed to **bypass the liver**, but they still remain **less popular than injections or gels**.

Choosing the Right TRT Method

Every man's body reacts differently to **testosterone replacement therapy**, so finding the best method often requires **trial and adjustment**. Some men prefer **the convenience of injections**, while others may opt for **daily gels or long-term pellet implants**.

The **most important factor** is **working with an experienced doctor** who can monitor progress, adjust doses as needed, and ensure that TRT is both **effective and safe** over the long term. **Understanding the pros and cons of each option allows men to make an informed decision** that best fits their lifestyle and health needs.

The Pros and Cons of TRT – What to Consider

Testosterone replacement therapy (TRT) can be **life-changing for men with clinically low testosterone**, restoring energy, strength, mental clarity, and overall well-being. However, it's not a magic bullet—while many men experience **significant**

improvements, others may struggle with **side effects, improper dosing, or dependency on treatment**. Understanding the **pros and cons** of TRT is essential before committing to a long-term regimen.

The Benefits of TRT

- **Increased Energy and Vitality** – Many men report feeling **more motivated, focused, and physically capable** within weeks of starting TRT. Fatigue fades, making daily life and workouts more manageable.
- **Stronger Muscles and Reduced Fat** – Testosterone **promotes muscle growth and fat loss**, helping men regain **lean body composition and strength**. Combined with proper diet and exercise, TRT can **enhance physical performance**.
- **Improved Mood and Mental Clarity** – Low-T is linked to **brain fog, depression, and anxiety**. Restoring testosterone often improves **mental**

sharpness, mood stability, and emotional resilience**.
- **Restored Libido and Sexual Function** – Testosterone plays a key role in **sex drive and performance**. Many men experience a **renewed interest in intimacy and stronger erections** after starting TRT.
- **Better Bone Density and Heart Health** – Long-term TRT **supports bone health**, reducing the risk of fractures and osteoporosis. Some research also suggests **testosterone may improve cardiovascular health** when properly monitored.

Potential Risks and Downsides of TRT

- **Testosterone Suppression (Shutdown of Natural Production)** – Once a man starts TRT, his body **reduces or stops natural testosterone production**. This means that if he ever decides to stop treatment, **his natural levels may take months (or longer) to recover**—or may never fully return to baseline.

- **Possible Fertility Issues** – TRT can **suppress sperm production**, making it difficult for men to conceive naturally. Those looking to have children may need to explore **alternative treatments** that boost testosterone **without shutting down natural sperm production**.
- **Increased Red Blood Cell Count** – Testosterone stimulates **red blood cell production**, which can **thicken the blood and increase the risk of blood clots or high blood pressure**. Regular blood tests are needed to **monitor hematocrit levels and prevent complications**.
- **Acne and Oily Skin** – Some men experience **increased oil production and breakouts**, particularly in the first few months of treatment. This is due to testosterone converting into **dihydrotestosterone (DHT)**, which stimulates **sebaceous (oil) glands**.
- **Estrogen Conversion (Gynecomastia Risk)** – Some testosterone converts to **estrogen (estradiol)**, which can lead to **water retention, mood swings, or even**

breast tissue growth (gynecomastia)** if levels rise too high. Proper **dosing and monitoring of estrogen levels** can help prevent these effects.
- **Dependency on Treatment** – Once a man starts TRT, **stopping treatment can cause a sudden drop in testosterone**, leading to **fatigue, depression, and a loss of previous benefits**. This is why **TRT should only be started if truly necessary**, and under careful medical supervision.

Who Should and Shouldn't Consider TRT?

TRT is **a powerful tool**, but it should only be used by men who **truly need it**. It's best for:

- Men with **clinically low testosterone (below 300 ng/dL)** confirmed by multiple blood tests.
- Those experiencing **severe fatigue, muscle loss, mood issues, and sexual dysfunction** that haven't improved with natural interventions.

- Men who **understand the long-term commitment** and are willing to monitor their health regularly.

However, TRT may **not be the best option** for:

- Men with **mild testosterone decline who haven't tried natural solutions first**.
- Those looking for **a quick fix without making lifestyle changes**.
- Men with certain **pre-existing conditions (such as untreated high blood pressure or severe clotting disorders)** without medical clearance.

Final Thoughts on TRT

TRT can be **life-changing**, but it's not a decision to take lightly. It requires **careful consideration, ongoing medical monitoring, and a commitment to long-term hormone management**. For those who truly need it, **the benefits can be immense**—but for those with **borderline Low-T or lifestyle-related testosterone decline, natural interventions should always be**

explored first before committing to lifelong treatment.

How TRT Affects Fertility and Natural Hormone Production

One of the most overlooked aspects of testosterone replacement therapy (TRT) is **its impact on fertility**. Many men start TRT without realizing that **exogenous (external) testosterone can suppress natural sperm production**, sometimes leading to **temporary or even permanent infertility**. Understanding how TRT affects the body's hormone system is crucial for those considering treatment—especially men who plan to have children in the future.

How TRT Shuts Down Natural Testosterone Production

The body regulates testosterone production through a **feedback loop involving the brain, testes, and pituitary gland**. When external testosterone is introduced through TRT, the brain **detects high testosterone levels** and signals the pituitary gland to **stop** producing **luteinizing hormone (LH) and follicle-stimulating hormone (FSH)**—the hormones that stimulate **natural testosterone and sperm production** in the testes.

Without these signals:

- **The testes stop producing testosterone**, leading to shrinkage over time.
- **Sperm production slows down or stops entirely**, causing reduced fertility.
- **The body may take months (or longer) to recover natural testosterone production if TRT is discontinued**.

For men who want to maintain **fertility while optimizing testosterone**, there are alternative approaches that can **boost testosterone without shutting down natural hormone production**.

Medications That Preserve Fertility While Boosting Testosterone

Instead of TRT, some men opt for **medications that stimulate the body's natural production of testosterone** while keeping sperm production intact. These include:

- **Clomid (Clomiphene Citrate)** – A selective estrogen receptor modulator (SERM) that stimulates the brain to **increase natural LH and FSH production**, boosting both testosterone and sperm count.
- **hCG (Human Chorionic Gonadotropin)** – Mimics LH, signaling the testes to produce **both testosterone and sperm**, making it a preferred option for men wanting to maintain fertility.
- **Enclomiphene** – A newer version of Clomid that specifically increases **LH and testosterone without affecting estrogen as much**, often leading to better results with fewer side effects.

These medications can be used **alone or in combination with TRT** for men who want the benefits of testosterone optimization **without the fertility risks**.

Can Fertility Be Restored After TRT?

For men who have already started TRT but want to restore fertility, **post-cycle therapy (PCT) can help restart natural hormone production**. This usually involves **hCG and Clomid** to stimulate LH and FSH and encourage the testes to **resume sperm production**. However, the timeline for recovery varies:

- Some men **recover within months** after stopping TRT.
- Others may take **a year or longer**, depending on how long they've been on TRT.
- In rare cases, **natural testosterone and sperm production may never fully return**, requiring ongoing medical support.

Final Considerations: TRT and Long-Term Hormonal Health

Before starting TRT, men should **weigh the benefits against the risks**, especially if they plan to have children. For those looking for **a fertility-friendly way to boost testosterone**, exploring **natural methods and medical**

alternatives like Clomid or hCG can be a smarter first step.

For those who do choose TRT, **being proactive about monitoring hormone levels, fertility markers, and overall health** is essential for making informed long-term decisions. The key is **working with a knowledgeable doctor** who understands both **testosterone optimization and fertility preservation** to ensure the best possible outcome.

Medications That Boost Testosterone Without TRT

For men experiencing symptoms of Low-T but wanting to avoid the potential downsides of **testosterone replacement therapy (TRT)**—such as dependency, fertility suppression, and hormone shutdown—there are **alternative medications that can naturally stimulate testosterone production**. These options help the body **increase its own testosterone levels**rather than relying on external sources.

1. Clomid (Clomiphene Citrate)

Originally developed as a fertility medication, **Clomid works by stimulating the brain's natural production of testosterone**. It blocks estrogen receptors in the hypothalamus, which tricks the body into producing **more luteinizing hormone (LH) and follicle-stimulating hormone (FSH)**—both of which are essential for testosterone production.

Pros:

- **Maintains fertility** while boosting testosterone.
- **Does not shut down natural testosterone production.**
- Can be an **effective first-line treatment for younger men with Low-T**.

Cons:

- May take **a few weeks** to notice effects.
- Can sometimes cause **mood swings or mild vision disturbances** in rare cases.
- Works best in men whose Low-T is **caused by secondary hypogonadism (a**

signaling issue in the brain rather than testicular failure).

2. Enclomiphene (An Improved Version of Clomid)

Enclomiphene is a **refined version of Clomid** that primarily works on increasing **LH and testosterone without affecting estrogen levels as much**. Some men experience **fewer side effects** with enclomiphene compared to Clomid.

Pros:

- Provides a **more direct boost to testosterone** than Clomid.
- **Less impact on estrogen balance**, reducing the risk of mood swings.
- Can be taken **orally with no injections needed**.

Cons:

- Not as widely prescribed as Clomid, meaning **availability may be limited**.
- May require **consistent blood work to fine-tune dosing**.

3. hCG (Human Chorionic Gonadotropin)

hCG is a **synthetic version of luteinizing hormone (LH)**, which **stimulates the testes to produce more testosterone naturally**. It is often used in combination with TRT to **prevent testicular shrinkage and maintain sperm production**, but it can also be used as a standalone therapy for men wanting to **boost testosterone without shutting down natural function**.

Pros:

- **Directly stimulates the testes to produce testosterone**.
- Helps **preserve fertility and sperm production**.
- Can be used **alone or alongside TRT** for men needing both approaches.

Cons:

- Requires **injections**, which some men may not prefer.
- **Higher costs** compared to oral medications like Clomid.
- Needs **regular monitoring** to avoid excessive estrogen conversion.

4. DHEA (Dehydroepiandrosterone)

DHEA is a **precursor hormone that the body converts into testosterone and other androgens**. Some men with Low-T **have low DHEA levels**, and supplementing with DHEA can provide a **small boost to testosterone**.

Pros:

- Available **over the counter** in many countries.
- Supports **hormonal balance and adrenal function**.
- Works **best in older men or those with adrenal-related hormone imbalances**.

Cons:

- **Effects are mild compared to other options**.
- Can convert into **estrogen if taken in excess**, requiring careful dosing.

Choosing the Right Approach

For men with **mild to moderate testosterone deficiency**, these medications can be a **good alternative to full TRT**, allowing the body to **continue producing its own testosterone** while improving energy, libido, and mental clarity.

However, **not all men respond the same way**, and blood work is essential to **track progress and ensure hormone levels remain balanced**. The right approach depends on **the cause of Low-T, personal health goals, and the need to preserve fertility**.

By exploring **natural hormone-stimulating options before jumping into TRT**, men can often achieve **optimal testosterone levels with fewer long-term risks and greater flexibility** in managing their health.

The Importance of Ongoing Monitoring and Adjustments

Testosterone therapy—or any medical intervention for Low-T—is not a **set-it-and-forget-it solution**. Whether a man is on **TRT, Clomid, hCG, or any other testosterone-boosting treatment, regular monitoring is**

essential to ensure **hormone levels stay balanced and side effects are minimized**.

Testosterone interacts with **multiple systems in the body**, including **blood circulation, metabolism, and even mood regulation**. If levels are too high or too low, unwanted effects can occur. This is why blood work and **adjustments to dosage and treatment plans** are necessary over time.

Key Blood Tests for Men on TRT or Other Hormone Therapies

Regular lab testing helps ensure **testosterone is at an optimal level** while preventing potential complications. The most important tests include:

- **Total and Free Testosterone** – Measures overall and bioavailable testosterone levels.
- **Estrogen (Estradiol, E2)** – Monitors how much testosterone is converting into estrogen, which can lead to **water retention, mood swings, or**

gynecomastia (breast tissue growth)** if too high.
- **Hematocrit and Hemoglobin** – Checks for **thickened blood**, which can increase the risk of high blood pressure and clotting.
- **SHBG (Sex Hormone-Binding Globulin)** – Determines how much testosterone is being **bound and inactivated in the bloodstream**.
- **LH and FSH** (if not on TRT) – Helps identify whether the body is still **producing its own testosterone** or if natural production has shut down.
- **Prolactin** – Elevated levels may indicate **pituitary gland dysfunction**, which can interfere with testosterone production.

Common Issues That Require Adjustments

Even when following **a well-planned treatment protocol**, some men experience issues that require **changes in dosage, frequency, or additional medications**. Common concerns include:

- **Excessive Estrogen Conversion** – If testosterone converts too much into

estrogen, symptoms like **bloating, mood swings, and water retention** can occur. This is usually managed by **adjusting the TRT dose or using aromatase inhibitors if needed**.
- **Fluctuating Energy Levels** – Some men feel great for a few days after an injection but **crash before the next dose**. Switching to **smaller, more frequent injections** can help stabilize levels.
- **Thickened Blood (High Hematocrit)** – Elevated testosterone can cause the body to **produce too many red blood cells**, increasing the risk of cardiovascular problems. If this occurs, doctors may recommend **lowering the dose or donating blood regularly to keep levels in check**.
- **Low Sperm Count and Fertility Issues** – If maintaining fertility is a priority, adjustments like **adding hCG alongside TRT** may be necessary.

Why Long-Term Monitoring Matters

Testosterone therapy is **not a short-term fix**—it's a **long-term health commitment**. What works at the start of treatment may need **adjustments over time**, depending on how the body responds.

By **monitoring blood work, tracking symptoms, and working with a knowledgeable doctor**, men can ensure their **testosterone remains in an optimal range**, maximizing the benefits of treatment **while minimizing risks**.

The key to success is **regular check-ins, making informed adjustments, and staying proactive about overall health**. With the right approach, testosterone therapy can be a **powerful tool for maintaining energy, strength, and vitality throughout life**.

Chapter 6: Regaining Vitality – A Long-Term Plan for Optimal Testosterone

How to Maintain Testosterone Levels Over Time

Boosting testosterone isn't just about **fixing a problem once—it's about maintaining long-term hormonal balance**. Whether a man has naturally restored his levels through **lifestyle changes** or is on **TRT or hormone-supporting medications**, the goal is to **keep testosterone optimized for life**.

Testosterone levels **fluctuate due to stress, diet, sleep, and overall health**, so maintaining high energy, strength, and motivation requires **ongoing effort**. Even men with naturally high testosterone can experience declines if they **ignore key lifestyle factors**.

The foundation of long-term testosterone maintenance includes:

- **Prioritizing Strength Training – Lifting weights at least 3–4 times per week**

keeps testosterone production strong and prevents muscle loss.
- **Eating Nutrient-Dense Foods** – A **diet rich in protein, healthy fats, and essential vitamins** supports testosterone synthesis and overall metabolic function.
- **Managing Stress and Cortisol** – Chronic stress **kills testosterone production**, so effective stress management is critical for long-term success.
- **Getting Quality Sleep** – Since most testosterone is **produced during deep sleep**, maintaining **7–9 hours per night** is one of the easiest ways to keep levels optimized.
- **Avoiding Environmental Toxins** – Limiting exposure to **BPA, phthalates, and processed foods** helps prevent hormone disruption.

When to Check Testosterone Levels

Even if symptoms improve, **periodic blood work is essential** to track testosterone levels and detect any **early signs of decline**. Most men benefit from testing **every 6–12 months** to ensure:

- **Testosterone remains in the optimal range** (not just "normal," but truly optimized).
- **Estrogen, cortisol, and other hormone levels stay balanced**.
- **Lifestyle adjustments are working**, and no medical interventions are needed.

Men who stay proactive about **monitoring and maintaining their testosterone levels** will find that **energy, muscle strength, mental clarity, and libido stay high well into later years**.

By treating testosterone optimization as **a lifelong strategy rather than a one-time fix**, men can **regain and sustain the vitality they deserve**, feeling their best for decades to come.

Why Tracking Progress Is Essential

When it comes to optimizing testosterone levels, **what gets measured gets managed**. Many men make the mistake of assuming that once they improve their testosterone—whether through **natural methods or**

medical treatment—they don't need to monitor it anymore. However, testosterone levels can **fluctuate over time**, and without tracking progress, it's easy to miss **early warning signs of decline**.

Regular tracking helps ensure that:

- **Testosterone stays in the optimal range**, rather than just the "normal" range.
- **Symptoms remain under control**—even if lab numbers look good, energy levels, mood, and strength are key indicators of hormonal health.
- **Adjustments can be made early** before testosterone levels dip too low or become too high.

How to Track Testosterone and Overall Health

Men who are serious about long-term hormonal balance should keep an eye on:

- **Blood Tests Every 6–12 Months** – Checking **total and free testosterone**, along with related markers like

estradiol, SHBG, and hematocrit, helps maintain proper balance.
- **Physical Performance and Recovery** – Strength, endurance, and how quickly the body **recovers from workouts** are direct indicators of testosterone levels.
- **Mental Clarity and Mood** – Testosterone plays a **huge role in motivation, focus, and emotional stability**. If brain fog, anxiety, or irritability increases, it may signal a hormonal imbalance.
- **Libido and Overall Drive** – A healthy testosterone level **supports a strong libido and ambition in all areas of life**. A sudden drop in these areas can indicate falling levels.

By keeping track of **both lab markers and physical symptoms**, men can take **proactive steps** to maintain high testosterone levels and prevent future issues. **The goal isn't just to boost testosterone—it's to sustain optimal levels for life.**

Creating a Sustainable Routine for Long-Term Health

Testosterone optimization isn't just about **fixing an imbalance**—it's about creating a **lifestyle that continuously supports hormone health**. Many men see short-term improvements but struggle to **maintain high testosterone levels over the long run**. The key is **building a routine that naturally keeps testosterone high**, without the constant need for drastic changes.

A **sustainable approach** means finding the right balance between:

- **Exercise and recovery** – Strength training is critical for maintaining testosterone, but **overtraining without proper rest can have the opposite effect**. A sustainable routine includes **resistance training 3–5 times per week**, combined with **active recovery days** to avoid burnout.
- **Nutrient-dense eating habits** – Testosterone thrives on **healthy fats, proteins, and micronutrients**. A long-term diet should include **whole, unprocessed foods** while limiting sugar,

processed seed oils, and artificial additives that disrupt hormone balance.
- **Consistent sleep patterns** – Men who maintain **high-quality sleep schedules** over time experience **better testosterone regulation, improved energy, and sharper cognitive function**.
- **Managing stress for hormonal balance** – Whether through **meditation, breathwork, outdoor time, or simple relaxation techniques**, keeping cortisol levels in check **prevents testosterone suppression**.

The **goal isn't to follow a short-term testosterone-boosting program**—it's to create a lifestyle that **naturally supports optimal hormone production year after year**.

Why Small, Daily Habits Matter More Than Quick Fixes

Many men **look for fast solutions** when dealing with Low-T, but the truth is that **hormone balance is built through**

consistent habits, not temporary fixes. The men who maintain **high testosterone levels into their 40s, 50s, and beyond** aren't necessarily doing extreme protocols—they're simply following **a structured, sustainable lifestyle** that works with their body.

By focusing on **long-term habits rather than quick fixes**, men can **stay energized, strong, and mentally sharp**—not just for a few months, but for life.

Combining Natural and Medical Approaches for Best Results

When it comes to maintaining **optimal testosterone levels**, the most effective strategy is often a **combination of natural and medical approaches**. While **lifestyle factors like diet, exercise, sleep, and stress management** form the foundation of hormonal health, some men may still require **medical interventions to reach or sustain their ideal levels**. The key is finding the right balance—**leveraging natural habits while** using medical support only when necessary.

Who Can Benefit from a Combination Approach?

- **Men with borderline Low-T** who have improved symptoms through **lifestyle changes** but still struggle with energy, libido, or muscle maintenance.
- **Older men experiencing age-related testosterone decline** who want to preserve their strength and vitality without completely shutting down natural production.
- **Men on TRT looking to optimize overall health**, ensuring their lifestyle supports their treatment rather than relying solely on medication.
- **Those who want to maintain fertility while increasing testosterone**, using alternatives like **hCG or Clomid instead of full TRT**.

How to Integrate Both Approaches Effectively

1. **Maximize Natural Testosterone First** – Before turning to medication, men should **optimize their diet, training, sleep, and stress management**. Even those on TRT will see **better results** when these factors are in check.

2. **Monitor Hormone Levels Regularly** – Whether using natural or medical approaches, keeping track of **testosterone, estrogen, and other key markers** ensures that treatment stays **effective and safe** over time.

3. **Use Medical Support Only When Necessary** – For some men, TRT or medications like **Clomid or hCG** may be needed, but they should be **strategically integrated** rather than used as a shortcut.

4. **Stay Flexible and Adjust as Needed** – Testosterone optimization is **not static**. Hormones shift based on **lifestyle, aging, and health changes**, so the best approach is one that **adapts over time**.

By combining **the best of both worlds**, men can experience **higher energy, sharper mental clarity, and stronger physical performance** without unnecessary risks. The goal is **not just raising testosterone, but optimizing overall health for the long run**.

The Future of Testosterone Research and Treatments

As science continues to evolve, the understanding of **testosterone, hormone optimization, and aging** is advancing at a rapid pace. What was once considered an inevitable decline in male vitality is now being challenged by **emerging research and innovative treatments**. The future of testosterone therapy and natural optimization looks promising, with new developments in **medical treatments, lifestyle interventions, and personalized health strategies** shaping the way men manage their hormone health.

Emerging Trends in Testosterone Research

- **Personalized Hormone Optimization** – With advancements in **genetic testing and precision medicine**, men can now get **highly individualized testosterone treatment plans** based on their **unique genetic and metabolic profiles**. This means **more accurate dosing and better results with fewer side effects**.
- **Safer, More Effective TRT Methods** – Newer formulations of **oral testosterone, long-acting injections, and bioidentical hormone therapy** are being developed to provide **more stable testosterone levels with fewer risks**.
- **Selective Androgen Receptor Modulators (SARMs)** – While still under research, SARMs are being explored as a way to **stimulate muscle growth and enhance testosterone function** without the full shutdown of natural hormone production seen in traditional TRT.
- **Peptides for Hormone Regulation** – Peptides like **Kisspeptin-10 and Gonadorelin** are being studied for their ability to **stimulate natural testosterone production**, potentially

offering an alternative to **TRT for younger men or those who want to maintain fertility**.
- **Testosterone and Longevity Science** – New studies suggest that **optimal testosterone levels may be linked to better cardiovascular health, brain function, and longer lifespan**, challenging the outdated belief that testosterone replacement increases heart disease risk.

What This Means for Men Looking to Optimize Testosterone

As more research emerges, men will have **more options and better tools** for maintaining testosterone levels safely and effectively. The key takeaway is that **testosterone optimization is no longer just about aging—it's about performance, vitality, and long-term health**.

By staying informed and **adapting to new scientific advancements**, men can continue to **feel stronger, more energized, and mentally sharper** well into later years. **The** future of testosterone therapy isn't just about replacement—it's about **full-spectrum hormone optimization that enhances overall well-being.**

Final Encouragement: Reclaiming Energy, Strength, and Confidence

Testosterone is more than just a number on a lab test—it's a **vital hormone that influences energy, motivation, strength, and overall quality of life.** While declining testosterone has been widely accepted as an unavoidable part of aging, the truth is **men have more control over their hormone health than ever before.**

Whether through **natural methods, medical interventions, or a combination of both**, optimizing testosterone is about **taking charge of your health, regaining vitality, and refusing to settle for low energy, brain fog, or reduced physical performance.**

The Power of Proactive Health Choices

Every man's journey to hormonal optimization will be different, but the most important factor is **staying proactive**. The key to long-term success is **not just fixing Low-T—it's maintaining a lifestyle that keeps testosterone levels high and ensures overall well-being**.

Men who take the time to:

- **Prioritize strength training, sleep, and nutrition**
- **Manage stress and limit environmental hormone disruptors**
- **Monitor hormone levels and make adjustments as needed**
- **Stay informed on the latest research and medical advancements**

Will continue to experience **stronger bodies, sharper minds, and more fulfilling lives** as they age.

You Have More Control Than You Think

No matter where you are in your testosterone journey—whether you're just starting to notice symptoms or already exploring treatment options—**there is always a way forward**. The information in this book provides the foundation, but it's up to you to **take action, apply what you've learned, and make choices that support long-term health and performance**.

By **investing in your hormonal health today**, you're setting yourself up for a future of **sustained energy, strength, confidence, and vitality**. Testosterone may naturally decline with age, but with the right approach, **you can stay at your best for decades to come**.

Printed in Dunstable, United Kingdom